ANGER MANAGEMENT: NEVER EXPLODE AGAIN!

A POWERFUL 3-STEP GUIDE AND WORKBOOK TO QUICKLY ANALYZE, UNDERSTAND AND DISSOLVE YOUR ANGER

ZARMINA PENNER

WWW.ZARMINAPENNER.COM

"All science is nothing more than the refinement of everyday thinking."

— ALBERT EINSTEIN

CONTENTS

I dedicate this book to my coaching clients, who have taught me so much about the intricacies of life.

A FREE GIFT FOR OUR READERS

To best prepare for the book, use this guide to identify your anger triggers quickly!

Just scan the QR code below!

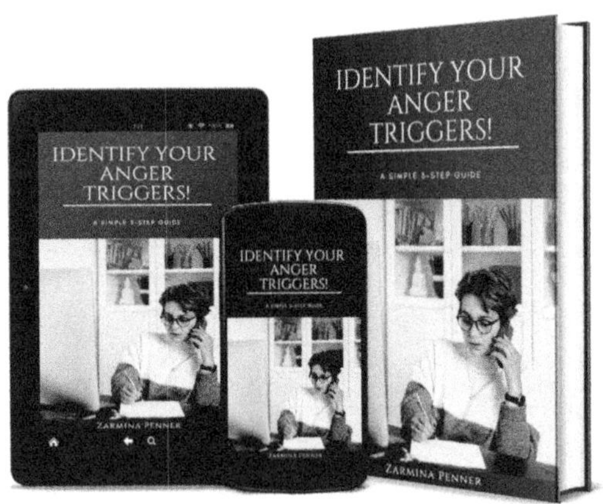

INTRODUCTION

"When anger arises, think of the consequences."

— *CONFUCIUS*

"You have an anger problem," they said, and you did not want to accept it for years. You pointed at others and their behavior to validate your right to be angry, and you tried to prove that you had been provoked. Besides, it's not good to suppress your emotions. So, you decided to let it all out. Something triggered you unexpectedly, and off you went.

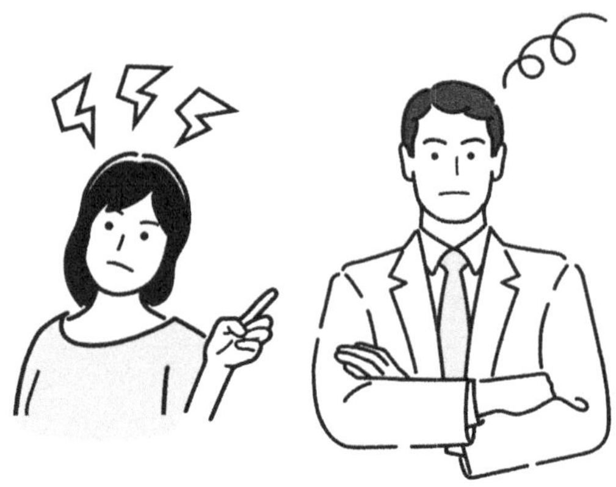

Image 1: You

However, your anger seems to be getting stronger with time and is showing up in situations that matter to you most. After many such incidents, you start believing that it might be true.

"Maybe I do have a problem..."

You've been searching for a solution that works. You've done your research, but the tips and tricks you have learned do not work once your blood starts boiling. It feels too late for control when you are figuratively standing beside yourself, overwhelmed by your anger.

If this is you, you are in the right place. This book exists for you. I assure you that anger is a widespread phenomenon, and you are not alone. Many of us struggle with anger, especially those who are passionate about our lives. I used to grapple with impulsive anger too. I can now confidently say that my anger is under control, and I look forward to signs of anger because I know they are just signs. Anger has become my friend, and hopefully, it will become yours too. Anger is merely a sign that something is not quite right, especially regarding boundaries, and we need to figure out what that is. Like other strong feelings, anger will point you to the path of self-development if you heed its call.

I am sure you will agree when I say that uncontrolled angry outbursts harm relationships. Since relationships are the basis for all we do and achieve in life, angry outbursts undermine our chance for happiness. They also undermine our success by ruining our reputations. Not only that, repetitive or prolonged anger wreaks havoc on our body chemistry. Because anger is part of our body's fight-flight stress response, it can keep us locked in a state of perpetual stress, which is certainly not healthy. Since you are here and reading these lines, I do not need to convince you that you need to manage your anger. You already know this.

Managing anger requires understanding why it is happening (your triggers) and how you react to it (your responses). Once you know, you must find ways to turn the situation around by changing your mind, outlook, and habitual responses. Turn things around by turning the downside into an upside. The upside, in this case, is that your anger is a clear sign that you need to fix something. Lashing out in anger contributes to the problem, not the solution, because others do not listen to angry people. Learning not to lash out gives you the luxury of choice to stop and reflect on what needs fixing.

We can be thankful for our anger, as it has a clear purpose. Finding the root cause puts you on an exciting journey to self-discovery, self-growth, resilience, and empowerment - to your true powerful self. Once you understand the underlying cause, you can devise a solution.

This book provides you with a simple three-step formula for anger management: The STOP! -1-2-3 Analysis and Solution Design. However, this requires some self-investigation and soul-searching in preparation, which takes time. Once you invest the time, your level of awareness will rise and place you at an enhanced starting point to address your anger more productively.

The first step to breaking the trigger-response-short-fuse cycle is consciously noticing the gap between trigger and response. A split second that you can become aware of and stretch out—knowing that you do not have to react. However, to use that split second in your favor, you will need prior mental awareness of your active triggers. You need to know why you respond in anger and devise a strategy for dealing with and controlling an anger incident. This preparatory work and paradigm shift helps you to not give in to your anger but instead work with it. You will even stop reacting automatically altogether in time.

I stumbled across a pragmatic solution by trial-and-error years ago while healing my anger impulses. During the past 20 years in my coaching practice, I have refined my mental Model, the STOP!-1-2-3 Model, and the process in order to better support clients. It is a model for self-analysis, the analysis of others, and the surrounding context. Working through the Model will give you a better awareness of yourself and others and higher situational awareness. You will undertake an autopsy of the incident and fully understand what, why, and how the anger incident happened. I speak from experience. Also, I want results. If a theory doesn't deliver, I discard it immediately to declutter my mind. Here I am offering you my distilled thoughts on anger management. Try my method out a couple of times and see if it works for you. Do not clog your mind with theories that do not work for you. This book will help you work through things, guide you to find solutions, and lead you to try new behaviors. Be hands-on and experimental. Reading alone will not be sufficient.

Before we move ahead, let me make two important distinctions:

Firstly, this book is about managing "garden variety" bouts of anger that negatively impact your life and relationships. *Oxford Languages Dictionary* defines anger as: "a strong feeling of annoyance, displeasure, or hostility." In contrast, it defines rage as "violent, uncontrollable anger." The difference between anger and rage is significant.

Anger may damage reputations and relationship-building, but it certainly has less potency than rage. Rage is a potential source of pain and destruction for oneself and others. It is closely linked with domestic and societal violence cases and means serious business.

If small triggers bring you, dear Reader, into a state of entirely mindless, highly emotional rage, this book may not be your complete solution. You will need more help. Full-blown rage incidents need therapeutic support, so consult with a trusted therapist. Similarly, if you are the receiver of extreme anger or rage from others, please take it seriously and quietly consult with a professional as early as possible. It's a crucial preventive step.

On the other hand, we will have those who do not or cannot feel their anger. For good reasons mainly based on childhood experiences, the conditioned mind does not allow them to tap into their anger (or potentially any other feeling). What they might notice instead of anger is a nagging sense of irritation after an interaction and, with time, a growing sense of resentment towards the other person involved for what they have to silently endure. If you, dear Reader, identify with this category, it is essential to establish a connection with your feelings first by respecting any emotion that does not feel good to you and sitting with it in silence. You will, with practice, slowly start to feel your anger (and other emotions) and move into the next stage of expressing yourself. At that point, this book will become relevant for you, too.

Secondly, I do not distinguish between genders, cultures, ethnicities, societal backgrounds, or other discriminators when managing anger. In terms of age, I am addressing anyone over 18—even better, 21. All other characteristics are irrelevant for anger management. If you often experience "a strong feeling of annoyance, displeasure, or hostility", this book is for you. You want to understand and manage this feeling better in order to improve your life and make your life more peaceful, productive, and successful. The book applies to everyone, but the examples in the book are workplace-oriented, where I have often used this process with my clients. My typical clients are over 30 years of age and in leading positions.

1

HOW TO USE THIS BOOK

> *"To ask the right question is half the solution of the problem."*
>
> — *CARL JUNG*

You can use this book as you would a workshop.

The introduction sets the scene, the scope, and the boundaries of this book. Then, we look at the mental model: STOP! -1-2-3. We will use this model to analyze and resolve anger incidents. You will examine yourself in a self-exploratory deep dive to build a refined foundation of thoughts about who you really are. Questions, checklists, and to-do lists will assist you in the process of self-exploration. Finally, a case study will illustrate the applied mental model and process for anger management.

Each chapter concludes with a summary, and you will find all the resources at the back of the book: links, question lists, checklists, and to-do lists. You can use these indefinitely to understand future anger incidents and gain more insight as you move ahead in your life.

The best way to work through this book is linear—chapter by chapter. Feel free to write in the spaces provided or anywhere you want to in the book. If you find the content helpful, make it yours and refer to it as often as necessary.

In parallel, I recommend using an app like Moodscope Lite by Hosford and Ashcroft (link in Resources section) to document your moods, triggers, and incidents while working through this book. It will open your eyes to what your current life situation is. I know from experience that such documentation can quickly pinpoint what is bothering you most. It is the fastest way to become consciously aware of what is happening to you on a daily basis.

Once you have completed the book, you should be able to:

- better know yourself and what you want
- better understand your current situation
- anticipate future incidents that could potentially trigger you
- stop automatically reacting to triggers
- see where you stand and what your next step could be
- use whatever trigger or incident that shows up to develop your awareness, sense of self, and resilience

Moving forward, train yourself not to be afraid of change. Move out of your comfort zone by constantly testing new insights and ideas. Take the time to move slowly and carefully adjust to them. Do not try to go the full mile too quickly, be strategic. You have all the time you need. Remind yourself regularly that your life is yours, and you can control it. When you go down a path with awareness, mindfulness, and self-knowledge, each subsequent best step will reveal itself to you naturally. That is a promise.

In summary, this book is here to inspire you in new ways while also providing you with a practical, effective, and straightforward method to deal with your anger challenge. I genuinely hope, dear Reader, it will give you a fresh start in dealing with others, especially when emotions run high.

2

UNDERSTAND ANGER

"Look deep into nature, and then you will understand everything better."

— *ALBERT EINSTEIN*

Paul Ekman[1] is a scientist who has done extensive research on human feelings and emotions, especially how they show up in facial micro-expressions. Ekman depicts seven universal emotions: anger, contempt, disgust, enjoyment, fear, sadness, and surprise. He sees anger as one of the most potent emotions and maintains that anger's primary message is simply, "get out of my way!"

David R. Hawkins[2] differentiates between negative feelings of shame, guilt, apathy, sadness, fear, lust, anger, or pride and positive feelings of courage, neutrality, usefulness, acceptance, reason, love, or peace. He examines the vibrations of each feeling and offers his view on how they may affect our thinking.

Theoretically speaking, there is much to say about anger and its various forms of expression. It can be complicated to understand and apply new learnings. In my practice with clients and my personal experience, I notice that anger arises most often when others do not respect us and our boundaries, and we deal with this by either suppressing or expressing our anger. Deliberately choosing to focus on expressed anger and boundary setting has helped my clients to manage their anger incidents faster, take control of their lives, and grow. This way, they can better deal with variations of their anger, even in the future. Setting boundaries gives us our chosen space. Those who irritate our spirit cannot gain access to our world, and the need for being in someone's face out of anger is reduced. Within these boundaries, we gain control of our lives and are now free to build up self-love, self-worth, and self-esteem. Once we have our stable footing and a peaceful life, we can expand our boundaries.

For example, I noticed that I expressed my anger very differently along my growth path. Initially, I suppressed anger which led to silent, simmering resentment under the surface. Then, I learned to express my anger and even enjoyed the feeling it gave me, which led to expressing my anger too often and suffering repercussions. Applying the three-step mental model and process as a shortcut to new insights, I now use my anger to self-reflect and respond consciously and intentionally.

In this book, I distinguish between feelings and emotions for clarity. *Oxford Languages* defines a feeling as "an emotional state or reaction."

Feelings are the first physical response to our thoughts. Feelings pass through our bodies if we process them correctly, much as clouds pass through the sky. If we do not process feelings and let them linger and fester in our bodies, they turn into emotional states that can negatively impact our mental and physical health, especially our immune system. The more intense the negative feeling, the lower your body energy level. Any strong emotion you repeatedly carry within yourself - not only anger - tells you it is undoubtedly time to bring your attention back to yourself, re-energize, reflect, and find out why.

Working with clients, I have noticed that emotional states of shame and guilt are often unconscious residuals of parental upbringing. Apathy and sadness can point to trauma, unprocessed grief, and self-repressive tendencies that keep us from living our lives fully. Lust, anger, and pride usually point to an over-active and under-managed ego-self. Anger points to potential boundary issues. We can struggle with one or multiple emotions at the same time.

Our goal in anger management is to move out of anger and both reach and remain in a stable upbeat feeling state, be it courage, neutrality, usefulness, acceptance, reason, or love, for as long as possible. The advantages are clear.

3

THE STOP! -1-2-3 MODEL

"Don't listen to the person who has the answers; listen to the person who has the questions."

— *ALBERT EINSTEIN*

As it turns out, everything relates to everything else. The more you analyze, the more ideas and insights you will have that seem relevant to the case. Discussion, then, compounds that with the opinions of others. Unfortunately, we tend to carry this information solely in our minds, which clogs our brains and hinders progress. This is the well-known analysis paralysis. Without a container for gathering and organizing your thoughts, anything you ponder deeply or discuss with others can, in time, turn into confusion.

I recommend using a pen and paper or a computer for a brain dump to de-clutter your mind. This is a highly relaxing activity.

The STOP! -1-2-3 model is a container for thoughts related to conflicts and emotional incidents, and provides you with an organized structure for analyzing anger incidents. These incidents usually relate to one underlying conflict. You will stumble across patterns that point you to the conflict by exploring different incidents. If you enjoy research, investigation, and training yourself to remain neutral, this process can be fun, and you will have "aha" moments that surprise you. You will also discover that you control more in your life than you initially thought.

HOW TO ANALYZE AN INCIDENT

The STOP! -1-2-3 Mental Model and Process: upper half and lower half

This mental model has two halves, i.e., two phases, for reflection:

1. Analysis: The upper half helps you to analyze the incident and underlying conflict in three steps.
2. Solution Design: The lower half helps you to design and tailor your solution in three steps.

It aims to move you swiftly and effectively through the analysis to the solution design and decision-making phase, as most issues remain in the analysis phase for far too long.

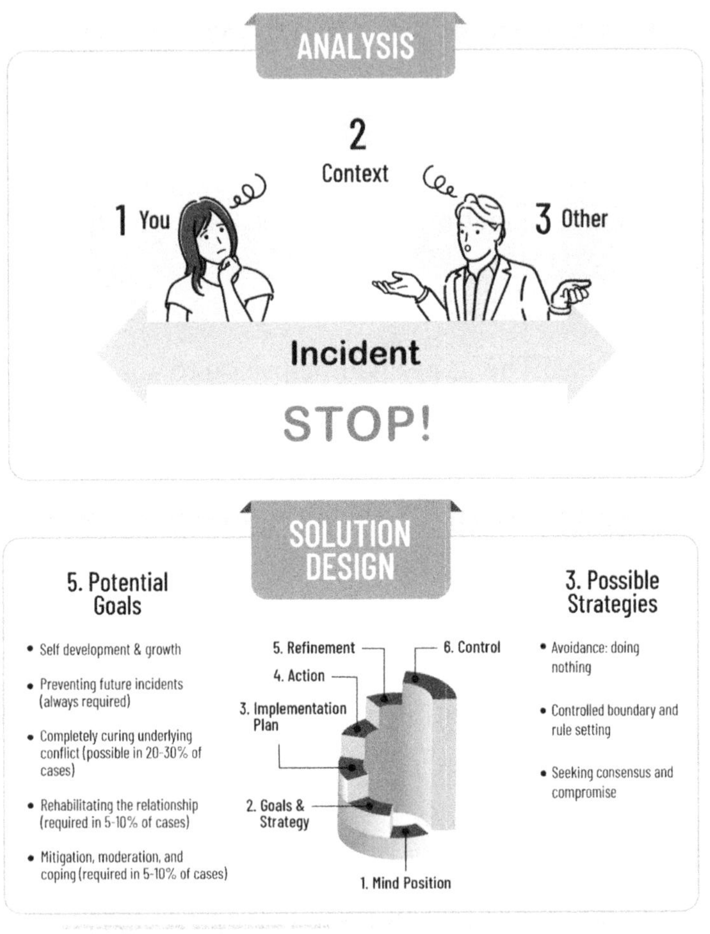

Image 2: The 1-2-3-Stop! Mental Model and Process: Analysis and Solution Design

Next, you will find the Analysis Tool (Phase 1) and, further along, the Solution Design Tool (Phase 2).

THE ANALYSIS TOOL

STOP! - 1-2-3, the upper half

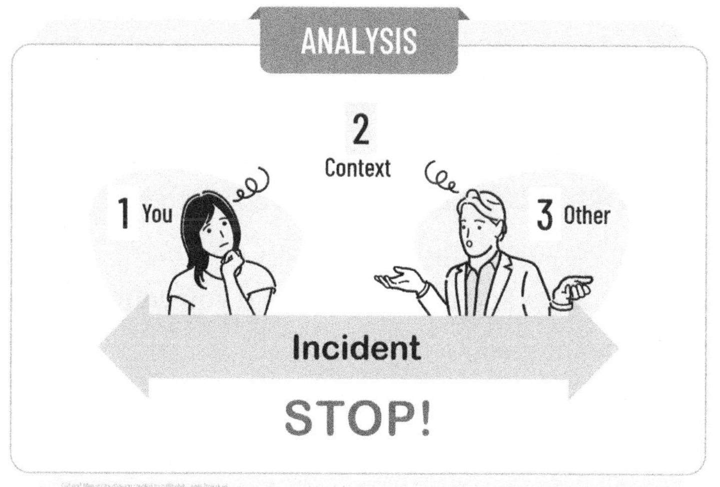

Image 3: The 1-2-3-Stop! Mental Model and Process: Analysis

Using the Analysis Tool

STOP! Stop and take some time to cool down before you do anything.

- Describe the incident, your response to the trigger, and the gap between stimulus and response. Pay attention to what you include and what you do not include in the story and how you tell the story. Take note if the story is about a victim and a perpetrator, and you depict yourself as a powerless victim. Notice how you feel about yourself and the other person. If you become very emotional, the incident may additionally link to memories of similar incidents with the same person or other persons not related to this incident.

- **You (1):** Read through what you've written in **STOP!** and extract whatever relates to you: the trigger, your feelings, and your responses. What did you do and not do? How did you contribute to the incident?
- **The Context (2):** Write down all aspects of the incident related to the context that might indirectly encourage such incidents. How did the context contribute to the incident? What are the enabling factors?
- **The Other Person (3):** Finally, write down how the other party contributed to the incident from your perspective. Also, include any intuitive hits you may have. The critical questions to ask yourself are: Does the other party respect you and your boundaries? How did the person or persons involved contribute to the incident? What does your gut tell you?

The tool helps us to avoid pointing fingers immediately at others, which is a natural tendency we must work to restrain. Notice that while analyzing, we do not go from the story of the incident (STOP!) straight to (3) the other party; instead, we take the longer route and explore the incident first (STOP!) and our contribution to it (1). Then we observe the context (2) and its contribution. The *last* step is thinking about others and their contribution. Teaching yourself to react in this manner is hugely advantageous and will promote self-growth and self-mastery.

You have now captured the incident well enough to consider a potential solution. To avoid analysis paralysis, train yourself to be satisfied with the knowledge you have. Knowing enough means having 80% clarity, because we can never know everything (100%) related to an incident. You will learn to recognize when you know enough to conclude the analysis with practice.

Let us apply the Analysis Tool. Here is the story of an anger incident (Example 1). This information goes under the STOP! Heading:

> *This morning, you had an incident at work with a junior co-worker and peer who produced a low-quality piece of input for your final paper. You know your co-worker well and had anticipated this incident*

> *two weeks ago at the beginning of the assignment. You had asked him to keep you in the loop and ask for help early enough. It is now Friday evening, and your deadline is Monday morning. You are still fuming because you know that your weekend plans just went down the drain; you will need to invest time over the weekend to produce the excellent paper you want to hand in to your boss. You do not want to miss your next promotion; this is a high-priority assignment.*

When he handed you his paper and went through it, you felt irritation and anger rapidly rise in your body. This added to the pressure you were already feeling about the final document, and there was no space left for empathy or tact. You told him exactly how you felt with a red face and a louder voice than usual. You reminded him of his agreement, but did not let him respond. Looking scared, he left quickly. Later you saw him huddled in a small group, apparently sharing what had happened. "Oh no, there goes my reputation!" you thought.

Example 1: Initial Overview

Underlying Conflict: *collaborating with a junior co-worker*

Context: *workplace*

Incident: *low-quality input for an important document*

People involved: *you, the junior co-worker, your boss, and those who observed the altercation or were told about it later*

Trigger: *a quality issue exacerbated by time and personal pressure*

Response: *anger, loud voice, aggressive behavior*

Under You (1): Look at yourself and your contribution to the incident. You had anticipated this happening, which means this is not an isolated incident. Knowing this, ask yourself:

- Did I establish respect, clarify expectations, and communicate my boundaries?
- Did I manage the process and the quality of the input well enough?
- Could I have given my co-worker another task, as the person responsible for the outcome?
- Could I have negotiated another contributor or a more flexible deadline with my boss?

Insights From You (1): This is an opportunity for growth and learning. All these aspects are on you and no one else. Do not let it happen again and learn from the experience as a leader.

Moving on to the Context (2): Because you had anticipated this happening, and it wasn't a one-off, there may be other contributing factors at play:

- Was there any follow-up after similar low-quality incidents in the past?
- Who is responsible for the individual development plan of your co-worker, and is this person aware of a quality issue?
- Is the process of creating high-quality papers well-thought-out in general? Is there room for improvement?

Insights From Context (2): Reflect on a tactful and productive way of addressing this issue with the person responsible for your co-worker—your boss. Touch on the general quality of the process first and your co-worker's role second. By doing this, you can potentially prevent similar incidents happening in the future.

Last, we look at the Other Party (3): Quality issues with junior co-workers are primarily caused by a lack of knowledge, skill, or experience. Assuming that this co-worker was suitable for the job and they harbored no ill-intent towards you, the questions you could ask now are:

- Is the co-worker willing to learn and confident enough to ask for help?
- Do they already have another high-quality skill you could use, i.e., how else could they contribute more effectively?
- Do they have an assigned coach or mentor to help them grow?

Insights From The Other Party (3): If you work together often, you could support your junior co-worker in his development by asking to be his mentor. An apology to the co-worker for your behavior and constructive feedback in a pleasant tone will show respect and understanding and control the damage. If your boss agrees, you could propose a mentoring plan.

When we pull these collective insights together, we can see the outline of a possible solution for current and possible future incidents and the potential to eradicate the underlying conflict entirely. Of course, this is an ideal scenario where all three aspects of the solutions (1, 2, and 3) can be implemented fully and fed into a continuous improvement process. In a less-than-ideal situation, you may not be able to change the impact the context has or have the opportunity to affect the other person directly. However, in any case, you always have the option to focus only on yourself and change your behavior. This is empowering as it gives you your power back.

There is one more piece of relevant information in this case. We established that the anger incident triggers were quality issues and time pressure. In addition to that, however, the incident seemingly links with your career and life path, well-being, and work-life balance. These overarching aspects make the trigger even more potent in your mind. The trigger was unconsciously complex because it related to other parts of your life, making it impossible for you to think on your feet and stay in control of your anger. It is easy to lash out at others, forgetting that our built-up pressure and heightened expectations may be the biggest contributing factor to the incident. Being clear about what you value in life and what is truly important will reduce complexity and help stop short-fuse anger explosions.

Concluding the analysis of this hypothetical case, we now have a quick and easy potential solution:

You (1)

- Prepare better and prevent this incident from happening again.
- Do some soul searching about your life plans to get more clarity and lower the pressure on yourself. Focus on well-being and health more than fast career progression.
- Notice and use the time gap between Trigger and Response. Resolve never to explode again.

The Context (2)

- Negotiate less time pressure with your boss.
- Ask to be the mentor of the junior contributor.
- Work with others to optimize work processes.

Other Party (3)

- Reduce the damage with an apology and an empathetic conversation with the co-worker. Clarify expectations and re-establish boundaries.
- Stop yourself from reacting by anticipating his behavior.
- Introduce humility, distance, and self-discipline in your behavior towards less qualified persons.

As you can see, this simple analysis process has already helped you to organize your thoughts. This pointed you roughly to the solution, step-by-step, before consulting the lower half of the tool: the solution design support. Now, we can refine our thinking process and the solution even more.

THE SOLUTION DESIGN TOOL

Remember, STOP! -1-2-3 is a complete model for analysis (the upper half of the illustration above) and solution design (the lower half).

In the lower half of the model, we carefully design the solution to the incident and its implementation. Well-rounded solutions have goals, a clear strategy, and a solution plan. There are five potential goals and three possible strategies for designing a solution plan.

Solution Design Tool: STOP! - 1-2-3, the lower half

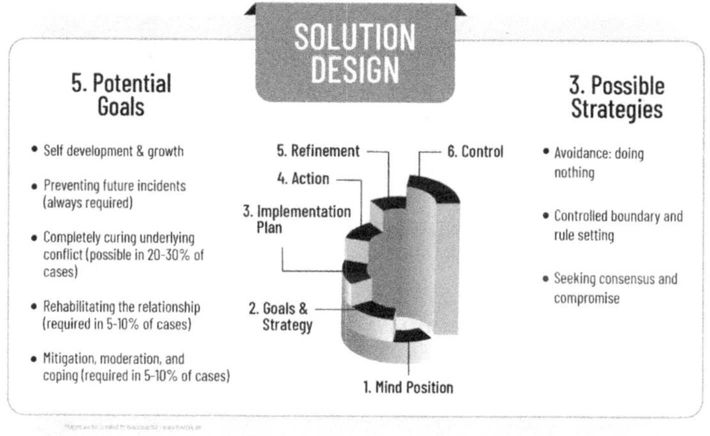

Image 4: The 1-2-3-Stop! Mental Model and Process: Solution Design

Once you decide upon the goals and your strategy, you will have the presence of mind and a steady foundation from which to devise your plan. You will not necessarily be able to resolve all conflicts and prevent all future incidents from happening, but you will have clarity.

Implementing, refining, and adapting your solution plan is essential until the dispute is manageable and under control. Each time you refine your solution plan, take a moment to re-think your goals and strategy because some aspects may have changed. We can only think so far ahead.

With your analysis findings, choose your Solution Goals (as many as you deem necessary) from the five potential goals depicted in the image. What do you want to achieve with the analysis findings and your learnings?

Then choose one solution strategy from the three possible strategies depicted in the image.

- Your Solution Goals:
- Your Solution Strategy:

Then design your Solution Plan:

- What is your position on this incident, your starting point?
- How will you implement your strategy and reach your goals? What are the first three steps you will take?

Let it sit for a while, and then take action. With each step, refine your plan of action. Your ultimate goal is to control the situation by behaving differently and preventing future incidents from happening. The lasting gift of the anger incident is the learning and growth you achieve from it.

Example 1: Case Summary

Underlying Conflict: *collaborating with junior co-workers*

Context: *workplace*

Incident: *low-quality input for an important document*

People involved: *you, the junior co-worker, your boss, and those who observed the altercation or were told about it later*

Trigger: *a quality issue exacerbated by time and personal pressure*

Response: *anger, loud voice, aggressive behavior*

Your Contribution to the Incident (1)

- *Not enough preparation*
- *Unclear values and priorities*
- *Potential lack of communication, process, and quality management, and not enough negotiation with your boss*

The Contribution of the Context to the Incident (2)

Context: *workplace*

- *lack of follow-up*
- *unclear responsibilities*
- *potential sub-par process*

Their Contribution to the Incident (3)

- *Lack of skill or knowledge*
- *Unclear picture of abilities*
- *Unclear development plan for the junior co-worker*

Solution Goals

- *Self-development & -growth: self-exploration for better awareness of self and situation*
- *Preventing future incidents (all cases): better preparation for such collaborations*
- *Completely curing the conflict (20-30% of cases): mentoring the junior co-worker*
- *Rehabilitating the relationship (5-10% of cases): a constructive conversation with the junior co-worker*

Solution Strategy

- *Seeking consensus and compromise*

Solution Plan

1. ***Position:*** *acceptance and humility*
2. ***Goals & Strategy:*** *4 chosen goals & consensus and compromise strategy*

3. ***Implementation Plan:*** *start next week*
4. ***Action:*** *meeting with the boss first*
5. ***Refinement*** *(WIP)*
6. ***Control*** *(WIP)*

4

UNDERSTAND WHO YOU ARE

"We cannot solve our problems with the same thinking we used when we created them."

— *ALBERT EINSTEIN*

Let us take our ongoing self-growth and development goal to explore and get to know ourselves better. Our findings will provide the backdrop we need to manage all future anger incidents and related conflicts. Clarity about ourselves and where we stand will significantly improve our ability to remain calm and collected in any situation, especially when we are angry.

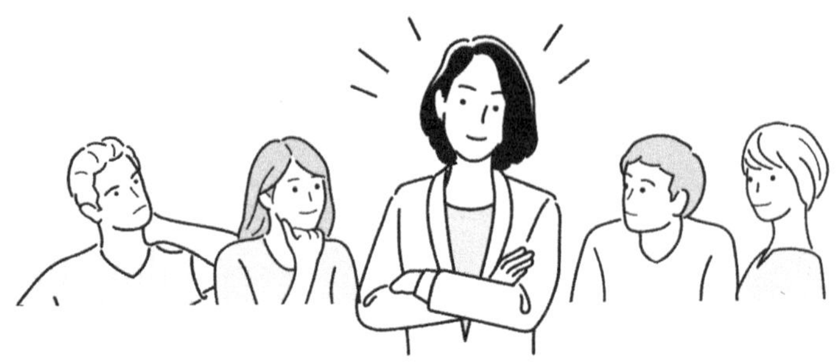

Image 5: The Unique You

THE UNIQUE YOU

Although the method for anger management is the same for everybody, the circumstances that make you angry differ. So, in order to understand your anger and find the best cure for you, you need to understand who you are, when and why you get angry.

To really know who you are, the concepts of identity, reputation, and personality are particularly helpful. According to Robert Hogan, identity is who you think you are, and reputation is how others perceive you.

Your Identity, Reputation, and Personality

- **Identity**

  Who you think you are
  Self-image
  A self-created concept
  To do: Brainstorm thoughts and beliefs about yourself

- **Reputation**

  How others perceive you
  To do: Take HOGAN Assessment (Flash Report). Ask for feedback from third party sources

- **Personality**

  Our consciousness boundaries
  To do: Take Test: Myers-Briggs-Personality Types (MBTI)

Identity is self-created; we can instantly change our minds about ourselves if we want to. It is our self-image and self-concept. We are the author, no one else. Simply put, we make our identity up in our minds. As

Carl Jung says: "The most important question to ask is: What myth am I living?"

For example, you may think of yourself as a quiet and generous person (identity). Others, acquaintances, or co-workers, may perceive you to be loud and stingy (reputation), especially those who haven't invested in getting to know you. How you may have behaved towards them in any random past interaction can lead to snap judgments on their part that are false. Their cloud of perception and conversations about you in your absence will impact your reputation, whether you like it or not. No amount of complaining will change these natural human tendencies in others. Since we cannot change others, we must manage perceptions to build a stellar reputation. Unfortunately, there is no way around it.

The gap between identity and reputation is where misunderstandings often arise and create opposing viewpoints that ultimately lead to conflict. Therefore, it is helpful to know the difference. We can reduce conflict potential by keeping our identity (self-image/self-concept) flexible and becoming mindful of the perception of others and our reputation. If others criticize us for being loud and stingy, we are less likely to become angry because we know it is their perception and not necessarily the truth. It will also give us data to work with: How did this perception come about? Am I unconsciously behaving in this way?

Hogan assessments measure probable reputation in the workplace using an extensive comparative database, with 95% accuracy. If you can get an evaluation through your organization, do so. It will tell you how others who do not know you may perceive you.

Fortunately, since everything starts with you, you can consider new ways of thinking and behaving to manage your anger better. If you so choose, you can change your identity in an instant. You may need to dig deeper, examine your underlying beliefs, and redefine them, but it really is possible. You may discover that a fixed identity (self-image/self-concept) based on pride keeps you from growing and maturing. It may also be contributing to incidents of anger when the ego-self flares up to protect itself.

As for reputation and the perception of others, know that your perception of yourself always weighs more. If you continue your self-examination and are open to feedback from those around you, the gap between identity and reputation will be minimal. Thus, there will be less potential for anger to arise in you.

Now let us talk about personality. Personality is the container for our ego-self. It is a product of nature and nurture in relatively equal proportions. Personality defines our consciousness and gives it boundaries. C.G. Jung proposes four psychological functions and two life attitudes to help us grasp the notion of personality:

- **Rational Function:** Thinking (T) and Feeling (F)
- **Irrational Function:** Sensation (S) and Intuition (N)
- **Life Attitude:** Introversion (I) and Extraversion (E)

To find out your personality type, take a Myers-Briggs-Personality test (MBTI) which builds on C.G. Jung's work. Some are free of charge (see resources for links to two test sites). Answer the test questions as authentically as possible and move swiftly through the test. It's best to take the test at different times: feeling relaxed and at peace, and feeling stressed and worked up. Compare the results. If they differ, read up on both personality profiles and reflect on them. Does the test result describe you well? You will find lots of information about personality types on the web.

Here are some quick and practical insights based on my observations of people and their personality types over the past 20 years. As you will see, each personality type reacts differently to triggers. If you have the following letters in your Myers-Briggs Profile, this is how you deal with stress and emotions, based on my observations.

Practical Insights about Personality Types Based on Observations

As mentioned above, C.G. Jung's Notion of Personality:

- Rational Function: Thinking (T) and Feeling (F)
- Irrational Function: Sensation (S) and Intuition (N)
- Life Attitude: Introversion (I) and Extraversion (E)

The Myers-Briggs Model also includes

- Outer World Orientation: Perceiving (P) and Judging (J).

Here are my observations about the Myers-Briggs types from my practice:

- **NF:** NFs are highly sensitive and easily overwhelmed by the emotions of others and the sheer amount of information they pick up with their senses. NFs tend to lash out (aggression) or repress emotions (depression).

- **SF:** SFs are feeling types that can become bogged down by details. SFs care about facts and remain fair to everyone; they are serious and hardworking.
- **NT:** NTs are highly analytical, quality-oriented, impatient, and can be controlling towards others; they tend to become irritated and angry quickly and might not handle emotions productively.
- **ST:** STs are highly analytical, not empathetic, and can be controlling towards others; they tend to become irritated and angry quickly, but might not show it.
- **P:** Ps are impulsive and do not like planning or making decisions. Ps do not like rules either.
- **J:** Js tend to be judgmental, critical of others and themselves, and do not react well to a change of plans; they can be controlling.
- **E:** Es are extroverted, outgoing individuals; they need people around them to re-energize. Being alone is stressful for them.
- **I:** Potentially shy individuals who need space, peace, and quiet to re-energize. Loud environments are stressful for them.

I have noticed in my work that it is perfectly normal for tests taken at different times - and on various test sites - to show different results. The test result taken in relaxed times will be closer to your genuine personality. The alternative one may describe your personality type under stress. For example, you might be an ESFJ (compassionate towards others) in a relaxed state, but when under pressure, you tend to move into an ESTJ state, with lower levels of compassion. Read up on both personality types, notice the shift, and train yourself not to react impulsively. Knowing the difference, and creating peaceful living and working conditions, will help you to stay in your original personality type. You can more easily access your gifts and talents in this mental space.

IN SUMMARY

- Let go of your current identity (self-image/self-concept) slowly to make room for the new you. Listen to how you talk about yourself to others and in your head. If you have a habit of saying, "I am a person who...", whatever it may be, stop. It may have been the case in the past, but it doesn't have to be in the future. Get out of the habit of theorizing, conceptualizing, and engage with life more directly. Let yourself feel your feelings and not react. You will feel less triggered in general. This will help you stay mindful and flexible in your outlook.

- Do a Hogan Assessment, specifically the so-called Flash Report, and get professional feedback on the findings. Once you know your behavior outliers, you can set up new behavioral guidelines for yourself. Practice them diligently. This effort will improve your reputation.For example, practice speaking more slowly and softly if others perceive you as too forceful and overbearing. In time, their perceptions of you will change.
- Know your MBTI personality type by reading up on it. Find and use your talents. There will be fewer surprises and confusion about who you are when you know yourself, and you can remain calm and collected during any anger incident.

These three self-explorative steps and a better understanding of yourself will reduce the potential for triggers to affect you emotionally. Your whole life experience will become more peaceful and satisfying.

You can do a lot to prevent anger by working on yourself, and you can transmute any problem you do not want in your life into a resilience-building and self-growth exercise. The secret is not to react when you feel angry. Using the split second between the trigger and the anger wisely can be utterly life-changing, helping you to not react but instead to respond constructively. When you're stressed, do not take yourself or your thoughts too seriously, and do *not* act. Any action at this time will prove to be out of place. Make sure you calm down first.

▶ Exercise 1

Your Identity, Reputation, and Personality

Describe your identity:

✎...

✎...

✎...

Describe your reputation, potentially with tests findings:

✎...

✎...

✎...

Describe your personality , with test findings:

✎...

✎...

✎...

5

UNDERSTAND WHAT YOU WANT

"Wherever you go, go with all your heart."

— *CONFUCIUS*

A feeling of satisfaction is the best indicator for knowing if what you want fits with what you have. Our feelings are vibrations in our body that signal unfailingly where we stand and if our path aligns with our values, i.e., what we want to have present in our lives. If you feel good and are satisfied, you are on the right route.

Persistent feelings of dissatisfaction are life's signposts that say "stop and reflect": Do you have what you value?

Those values differ for each of us. Common examples are inner peace, family, freedom of thought, financial freedom, security, knowledge, creativity, helping others, feeling connected, and being knowledgeable. There are many more, of course. To identify your values, describe the conditions that must be present in your life for you to feel satisfied. Those conditions are your values because you value having them present in your life. For example, if you value family life and freedom of thought, you might not want to work long hours in a hierarchical organization with rigid rules of interaction.

Values will change over time, so make a habit of doing this exercise at least once a year. Brainstorm, validate, and prioritize five values, keep them somewhere visible, and use them for making important decisions.

VALIDATION

We must understand where our values stem from; therefore, we must distinguish between the ego-self and the higher self. Valid values stem from the non-ego self, the higher self, not the ego-self.

Oxford Languages defines the ego as "a person's sense of self-esteem or self-importance." There is no definition there for the higher self in this dictionary. *Wikipedia* defines the higher self as a term linked with belief systems. It describes it as an "eternal, conscious, and intelligent being, who is one's real self." Such existential beliefs are very personal, and it is up to you, dear Reader, to decide if the concept of the higher self works for you. We must, however, distinguish between two states of mind, one of which is the wise one.

The ego-self tends toward selfishness, and we need to have controls in place to recognize its invalid values. Typical invalid values can be accumulating money, material belongings, and power at any cost. The wise non-ego-self prefers a solution where everyone benefits. It is the absolute opposite state of mind. If you feel compelled to do so, many books are available to help you dig deeper into the differences between the two mental states.[1].

Choose values that benefit you and others, as in "doing well while doing good". That is the most straightforward validation you need for your chosen values.

▶ **Exercise 2**

The Primary Five Values of Your Wise Non-Ego-Self

Value 1:

Value 2:

Value 3:

Value 4:

Value 5:

ASSESSMENT

Let us assess who controls your life right now: your ego-self or your non-ego self.

The ego-self has a perpetually negative outlook and sees problems everywhere, also in others. The ego is not an enemy, but it wants us confined and "safe" within a designated space—our so-called comfort zone. It doesn't want us to venture out; therefore, it tends to be both overprotective and fearful of change.

The ego-self also typically feels inadequate, incompetent, and in constant competition with others. Not wanting to feel the pain, the ego-self projects its thoughts of inadequacy and incompetency onto others. That's why we get mad at others - we see in them what we try to avoid seeing in ourselves (our blind spots). If our emotions toward others are powerful, then there is a high probability that the issues originate within us, and we project them onto others. Therefore, lashing out is never a good idea.

If we ground ourselves in our carefully curated and validated values and use them to vet our thoughts and feelings, we will slowly but surely move into calmer waters with our ego-selves in check.

Here is a test to assess who is in charge. Be diligent and work on this until you answer all twelve questions with a confident "no". If any of the following statements apply to you, you will still need to gradually dethrone your ego-self and hand the reins over to your wise non-ego self (higher self).

▶ Exercise 3

Ego-self test: Please evaluate with yes, no, or yes/no.

Statements that point to the ego-self running your life

1. *You are proud of yourself and your achievements; you frequently look down on others.*
2. *You talk over others and think you know all the answers.*
3. *You are envious of what others possess.*
4. *You tend to be judgmental and want to minimize the achievements of others.*
5. *You can quickly get angry and even go into a rage.*
6. *You have an underlying feeling of dread and anxiety. You have many fears.*
7. *You feel helpless and powerless to change your situation.*

8. *You feel guilty and think you are not doing enough.*
9. *You have low self-esteem. People can easily shame you and take advantage of you.*
10. *You feel despair and self-doubt, and you do not know your own worth.*
11. *You frequently complain about your life circumstances.*
12. *Others trigger you quickly, and you have frequent emotional ups and downs.*

As you can see, your ego-self may be the source of your anger problem—discerning between the ego-self and the non-ego (higher self) is therefore crucial. Ultimately, we want to become fully aware of how our unchecked ego-self sabotages our lives. The ultimate goal is to move our ego-selves into a healthy, intelligent, capable, and compliant version that helps implement the non-ego self's value-driven commands.

MEDITATION

Silent meditation is the most effective tool to support you in understanding and managing your ego-self and mastering your emotions.

Take 5 - 10 minutes every morning before the day starts, right after brushing your teeth:

- Listen to your ego-self's talk without engaging in it.
- Notice what your body tells you and where tension sits.
- Listen to what your gut, your intuition, tells you.

That is how you learn to respect your mind, body, and instinct and slowly regain control of your ego-self. With time, you will notice the difference between a negative thought of the ego-self and the inspired, uplifting thought of the wise non-ego self. There will be no uncertainty about which thought is the better guide in your life.

Reflecting on incidents of anger in your daily life, become particularly aware of the ego-self's tendency to project its perceived shortcomings onto others. Notice when your ego-self is again in the driver's seat. Pay attention, coach, and coax your ego-self into a more positive non-ego state of mind and reflect on the incident again, as described above.

For example, you may feel angry about someone procrastinating on a task. Notice your thoughts, but do not take them seriously and start nagging others. Look at the label you are giving the person—in this case, procrastinator—and ask yourself if and when *you* tend to procrastinate. Reflect. Heal your procrastination and then have a friendly conversation with the other person about a said task or find a different contributor.

You are teaching yourself to feel your feelings, not react, and you are training yourself to think and feel simultaneously. Managing the ego-self is a crucial component of anger management.

IN SUMMARY

- The best indicator for knowing where you currently stand is a feeling of satisfaction.
- Deal with dissatisfaction by asking yourself: what exactly do I want?
- Ask yourself first what you value and then ground yourself in those values.
- Then, take a closer look at your ego-self. Is it driving your life? If so, take away the control.
- Become aware of your ego-self projections onto others and train yourself to think and feel at the same time.

6

UNDERSTAND YOUR CONTEXT

"A man should look for what is, and not what he thinks should be."

— ALBERT EINSTEIN

We never operate in a vacuum; therefore, it is crucial to qualify your context. Whatever we do and experience depends on and relates to the context we have chosen for ourselves. The context may create conditions that lead to conflict and daily incidents, independent of who you are and what you want.

Prevention is everything when it comes to context. After careful research and consideration, if you realize that your context does not truly support your personality, values, and talents, choose one better suited to you. You may avoid many incidents of anger that challenge your peace of mind and quality of life. The objective is to know, accept, and work well within your chosen context.

Let us look carefully at three aspects of a context—culture, rules, and key players. Although this is not a comprehensive analysis, it is sufficient for our objective of anger management. With closer examination, you will better grasp how your context may contribute to your anger incidents and ongoing conflicts.

CULTURE

According to the *Hogan MVP assessment* (flash report), the leader's motives, values, and preferences influence workplace culture and the people who work within it. In my opinion, we can use the essence of this assessment to understand the culture of any setting.

You, as an individual, have your motives, values, and preferences, as well. If the two sets of MVPs - yours and that of your context - fit reasonably well together, you will be able to thrive in it. Otherwise, you will invariably run into situations that go against your grain and provoke your feelings, and potentially anger in you. It is as simple as that.

Below you will find HOGAN's list of motives, values, and preferences for a quick and easy analysis of your context (alternatively, take HOGAN's formal MVPI assessment). It is not available to the public, but your organization may have access to it. If not, it is still helpful to do a quick analysis here and identify any mismatch.

▶ Exercise 4

You and Your Context: Culture Assessment

Based on HOGAN's 10 MVPs (motivations, values, and preferences), evaluate the culture of your context. Answer with yes, no, or yes/no:

Recognition: being known, seen, visible, famous

- Do you value recognition?
- Do the leaders in your context value recognition?

Power: challenge, competition, achievement, and success

- Do you value power?
- Do the leaders in your context value power?

Hedonism: fun, excitement, variety, and pleasure

- Do you value hedonism?
- Do the leaders in your context value hedonism?

Altruistic: serving others and helping the less fortunate

- Do you value altruism?
- Do the leaders in your context value altruism?

Affiliation: frequent and varied social contact

- Do you value affiliation?
- Do the leaders in your context value affiliation?

Tradition: morality, family values, and devotion to duty

- Do you value tradition?
- Do the leaders in your context value tradition?

Security: structure, order, and predictability

- Do you value security?
- Do the leaders in your context value security?

Commerce: earning money, realizing profits, finding opportunities

- Do you value commerce?
- Do the leaders in your context value commerce?

Aesthetics: the look, feel, and design of products and artistic work

- Do you value aesthetics?
- Do the leaders in your context value aesthetics?

Science: new ideas, technology, and rational problem-solving

- Do you value science?
- Do the leaders in your context value science?

Identify where you see mismatched responses and then reflect on them.

Could the mismatch have led to any anger incidents you have experienced so far?

▶ **Exercise 5:** ***Your insights regarding your culture***

Now reflect on the comparison of the cultural values and summarize your findings:

- What mismatches do you see?

✎...

- What does this mean to you?

✎...

- *What are your insights and conclusions of the evaluation?*

✎...

RULES OF THE GAME

Secondly, we want to look at the "rules of the game" in your context. Whatever you do in your context, i.e., the "game" you participate in, will be governed by spoken and unspoken rules and regulations.

Challenge yourself to quickly brainstorm and prioritize ten rules that govern your context and reflect on how you feel about each of these.

▶ Exercise 6

Your Insights regarding Rules of the Game in your Context

Identify the apparent and hidden rules of the game in your context:

1. *What are the 5-10 rules in your context?*

✎...

✎...

✎...

2. *Which rules are acceptable to you?*

✎...

3. *Which rules irritate you and make you angry?*

✎...

4. *If so, is there a way to decrease the sense of irritation?*

✎...

5. What else do you notice?

✎...

6. What is your conclusion?

✎...

For example, you work in an organization that wants you to clock in on time, you, however, regularly miss the morning deadline. If so, you can reflect on what is preventing you from being on time and set up a routine that helps you adhere better to the rules. This is simple troubleshooting to clean up any contributors to anger incidents.

As you can see, we are not talking about changing others. We are constantly talking about taking responsibility for how things are and finding ways to grow and cope, thereby decreasing conflict potential and anger-inducing incidents.

KEY PLAYERS

In a third step, we want to brainstorm and identify your context's 5-10 key players.

▶ Exercise 7

Key Players

Identify the key players in your context:

Name the context:

- Who are the 5-10 key players who define your context?

✎...

✎...

✎...

- What are they passionate about? What do they value?

✎...

- What are their goals?

✎...

- Do these key players have a joint vision? What is it?

✎...

- What is your ambition in this context? Do you want to be a top player?

✎...

If you are operating in more than one context, do the three-step (culture, rules, and key players) exercise described above for each one.

IN SUMMARY

To know your context well, we need to look at three aspects: culture, rules, and key players.

We define culture using Hogan's ten motives, values, and preferences (MVP). Then we identify the "rules of the game" and finally analyze the key players and their aspirations. Once we do this and take appropriate precautions, we lessen the number of situations that could catch us off guard and bind the mind power we desperately need to think on our feet, feel our feelings, and make better decisions regarding behavior, and not react to triggers.

7

UNDERSTAND WITH WHOM YOU INTERACT

"Weak people get revenge, strong people forgive, and intelligent people ignore."

— *ALBERT EINSTEIN*

Your life revolves around the people you know and interact with on a regular basis. They may trigger you intentionally or unintentionally, and they may be privy to your anger incidents. Therefore, it makes sense to reflect on them.

Messy interactions lead to unnecessary conflicts and incidents, low-quality outcomes, and unclear relationships.

All interactions, no matter with which group, are made up of three parts:

1. preparation
2. execution
3. post-processing

The split remains the same in any context. In a work setting, interactions are more structured. Preparation roughly contributes 60% to the quality of the outcome of the exchange, execution 30%, and post-processing 10%, in my experience.

Each essential interaction, especially those with high stakes, needs to be well-prepared. This will support you in remaining calm and collected in execution. All kinds of issues can arise later if the preparation is not good enough.

In terms of preparation, it is most helpful to focus on:

- content of the interaction: the what
- goals: the why
- participants and their viewpoints: the who and for whom

Interactions need facilitation, and everyone needs to know their roles and responsibilities. There should be behavioral guidelines—implicit or explicit—for those participating in the exchanges, even in a 1:1 interaction.

Post-processing helps you to learn from the exchange. It is also a reminder for the participants of what took place and how they need to follow up.

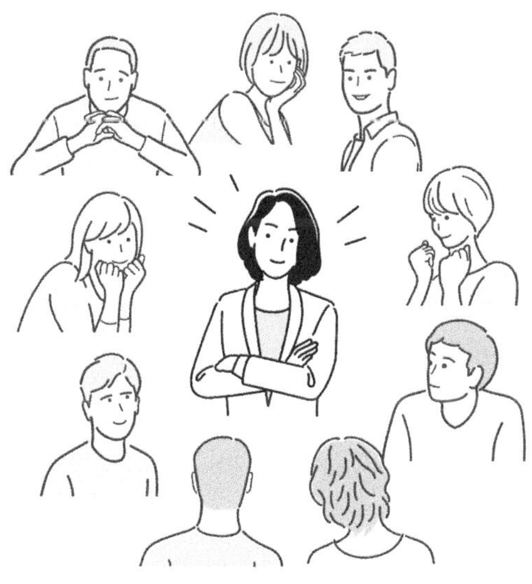

Image 6: The people you interact with

Take the people in the context you analyzed above.

1. Draw a circle on paper.
2. Place yourself in the middle.
3. Brainstorm the persons you interact with most and plot them around you.

Once you have identified them, copy their names into the table below and distribute them into the following four groups.

1. **The Indifferent:** No interaction or feelings are involved. This is a fringe person, like an extra in a show.
2. **The Neutral:** Most interactions are short service-manner transactions and encounters—no relationships.
3. **The Positive:** Interactions are uplifting, resulting in relationships and positive emotions.
4. **The Negative:** These confusing, draining interactions and complicated relationships result in negative emotions.

We label and discern to understand and improve interactions and relationships. This will also help us to anticipate anger-provoking triggers.

▶ Exercise 8

People you interact with regularly in the workplace

Identify the ten people you interact with most in your context:

Name the context:

1) Name of the person:

Indifferent (1), neutral (2), positive (3), or negative (4)?

2) Name of the person:

Indifferent (1), neutral (2), positive (3), or negative (4)?

3) Name of the person:

Indifferent (1), neutral (2), positive (3), or negative (4)?

4) Name of the person:

Indifferent (1), neutral (2), positive (3), or negative (4)?

5) Name of the person:

Indifferent (1), neutral (2), positive (3), or negative (4)?

6) Name of the person:

Indifferent (1), neutral (2), positive (3), or negative (4)?

7) Name of the person:

Indifferent (1), neutral (2), positive (3), or negative (4)?

8) Name of the person:

Indifferent (1), neutral (2), positive (3), or negative (4)?

9) Name of the person:

Indifferent (1), neutral (2), positive (3), or negative (4)?

10) Name of the person:

Indifferent (1), neutral (2), positive (3), or negative (4)?

THE OBSERVERS (INDIFFERENTS AND NEUTRALS)

I call the first two groups - the indifferent and the neutral - the observers. We frequently underestimate their impact on our lives. The observers are the backdrop for everyone else and potential supporters in need. This analysis will help you to become aware of them and remain mindful and appreciative when your paths cross. It is essential to maintain a gracious, authentic, and polite manner with them. This will serve you and them, as well as build your reputation. Observers who perceive themselves as less regarded will most definitely notice and appreciate you if you are mindful and polite toward them. It's vital to behave in the same cordial manner with everyone, no matter where you stand in terms of status in their context.

Interacting with the two last groups, i.e. the positive and the negative, is different because we have relationships, not just interactions. All relationships require a level of trust, respect, and also boundaries.

THE POSITIVE

In positive and uplifting relationships, remaining mindful is necessary. Why? Because we are emotionally attached, we usually have high expectations of their appreciation of us. If the other person doesn't respond as expected, this may send us to the valley of despair, and we may assume we have displeased them. Anger and resentment can follow. In this dynamic, we must avoid willingly handing over our power to them. Hanging onto our power and self-esteem while respecting them is an absolute must. This takes some practice, but if you master it, the most beautiful, harmonious, and respectful long-term relationships can emerge.

It is interesting to note that, backed by our admiration, we may project our positive sides onto them, and our feelings of respect toward them may skyrocket. In this case, ask yourself what you admire about these people. Know that you have seeds of whatever you admire about them in yourself; otherwise, you wouldn't have noticed the trait. If we stay mindful and aware, we can thrive in their midst and grow way beyond what we expect of ourselves.

THE NEGATIVE

For the same reason, be particularly cautious of the last group, the negative. They also serve as a significant source of potential growth, though it will take more precautions, mindfulness, and self-care to enjoy your self-development. The key to handling this group well is to master your emotions in order to remain immune to their pattern of actively triggering those around them to brandish their power.

We will now dig deeper into this group and analyze your active conflicts and related incidents.

8

UNDERSTAND YOUR ACTIVE CONFLICTS AND RELATED INCIDENTS

"Stay away from negative people. They have a problem for every solution."

— ALBERT EINSTEIN

To better understand the fourth group of people with whom you frequently interact (the negative group), focus on unresolved conflicts you regularly experience with them. List and describe them and prioritize the conflicts you want to resolve first by how intensely they affect your mood.

ANALYZE THE CONFLICT, THE ROOT CAUSE

▶ Exercise 9

Current active conflicts in this context

Directions:

1. Give each conflict a name, for example, *"Taker" Personality*
2. Who else was involved in this conflict? *Negative A, Observers B, C, and Positive D, E*
3. How old is the conflict? *One year*
4. How much does it affect your mood? *90%*
5. What are typical triggers in these incidents? *Asking for favors and not returning them*
6. What's the priority for resolution?

Now, identify your three currently active conflicts in this context:

Name the context:

Name of conflict:

- Name of the person involved:
- Are others involved?
- Age of conflict:
- Degree of Stress (Impact on Mood) in %:

- Typical Triggers
- Priority for resolution:

Name of conflict:

- Name of the person involved:
- Are they indifferent (1), neutral (2), positive (3), or negative (4)?
- Are others involved?
- Age of conflict:
- Degree of Stress (Impact on Mood) in %:
- Typical Triggers
- Priority for resolution:

Name of conflict:

- Name of the person involved:
- Are they indifferent (1), neutral (2), positive (3), or negative (4)?
- Are others involved?
- Age of conflict:
- Degree of Stress (Impact on Mood) in %:
- Typical Triggers
- Priority for resolution:

Each conflict can have multiple incidents. Choose the most recent incident and use the STOP! -1-2-3 model to analyze what happened, as we described above (Phase 1). Look for recurring patterns and educate yourself about the nature of the conflict and related incidents. Our goal is to be able to anticipate and avoid recurrence.

Here are some initial questions to get the juices flowing before you populate the Analysis and Solution Design Tool:

Describe the incident and tell the story.

1. In short, what happened?

✎…

2. Who was the other person? Who else was involved?

✎…

3. Was there a recurring conflict that led to this incident?

✎…

4. Was the matter related to trust, respect, expectations, and boundaries?

✎...

5. How did the interaction start?

✎...

6. What triggered your anger, and what was your response to it?

✎...

7. Did your response ease or exacerbate the situation?

✎...

8. What was your contribution to the incident?

✎...

9. What was the context contributing to it?

✎...

10. How did they contribute to the incident?

✎…

11. How did the interaction end?

✎…

12. How did you feel about it immediately afterward and now?

✎…

▶ **Exercise 10**

Analysis Tool: STOP! -1-2-3, the upper half

Now summarize the analysis findings:

- **Potential underlying conflict:**
- **Context:**
- **Incident:**
- **Your name:**
- **Their name:**
- **Others involved:**
- **Trigger:**
- **Response:**
- **Your contribution to the incident:**
- **The context's contribution:**

- **Their contribution:**
- **Significant details:**

DESIGN A SOLUTION FOR THE UNDERLYING CONFLICT

One conflict may lead to multiple incidents. So if it is not an isolated incident, dig deeper and try to find the underlying pattern, i.e., the root cause of the conflict. This way, you can prevent many future incidents from happening.

Focus on one conflict, resolve it, and slowly move on to the next—do not rush. Rinse and repeat for the prioritized conflicts and related incidents on your list. Later, search for new ones to consider. Make notes and track your insights and conclusions. This will help you to understand yourself and others better with each incident.

Solution Design Tool: STOP! - 1-2-3, the lower half

Choose your goals and strategy and design a solution plan:

Solution Goals

- **Self-development & -growth:**
- ***Preventing future incidents*** *(always):*

- **Complete curing of the conflict** (20-30% of cases):
- **Rehabilitation of the relationship** (5-10% of cases):
- **Mitigation, moderation, and coping (5-10% of cases):** *Keeping diplomatic distance from Boss and Team Member A*

Solution Strategy:

Solution Plan:

- ***Position:***
- ***Goals & Strategy:***
- ***Implementation Plan:***
- ***Action:***
- ***Refinement:***
- ***Control***

The good news is that interactions with groups three (Positive) and four (Negative) carry valuable learnings and growth. By educating yourself beforehand about the people in your life, you will anticipate incidents, triggers, and recurring patterns, remain calm, and maintain distance and mindful awareness while incidents occur. Careful analysis and solution design will move you slowly from feeling helpless and reactive into a proactive, responsible state of mind.

Again, I want to underline the aspect of safety, as I did in the introduction. Learning and self-growth are beneficial, but keeping yourself safe is critical. All potentially abusive relationships begin with so-called red flags, minor signs of things not matching up. Safety is relevant for all four groups. Train yourself to recognize if something sounds or feels off in peripheral interactions concerning groups one and two, the observers. Make it a habit to be aware and always trust your gut.

If you quickly add a newcomer to group three (positive relationships) and the relationship moves too fast, take heed. Watch out for those who do not want to take the time to build trust with you and shower you with overt signs of affection too early. If something feels too good to be true, it probably is. Use your power to think and feel simultaneously and remain observant for 9 to 12 months. Authentic, positive relationships and trust-building take time.

With Group four, train yourself to notice how they deal with conflict and your resolution offers.

Here are questions to ask yourself:

1. Are they earnestly considering your proposal(s) for a solution?
2. Do they listen carefully and respond?

3. Are they kind to you in both demeanor and words?
4. Do they respect you and your boundaries?
5. Do they accept responsibility for the incident or conflict?
6. Are they able to control their emotions?
7. Do they show remorse and try to change their ways after a conversation?
8. Does the interaction feel right? What does your gut feeling say?

If any answer is a no, you have a red flag.

Educating yourself about mental health, narcissism, and narcissistic personality disorders is a good idea, as it is essential life information[12]. Abuse can be covert or overt. A hallmark of abusive personal relationships is the on-again, off-again relationship cycle.

Do your conflict and incident analysis using the tools described above. Wisely choose your strategy and goals with Group 4. In extreme cases, opt to do nothing and move carefully out of their orbit. If you cannot leave, become aware of what is happening and relate to them only in safely curated transactions. Ensure you seek support.

IN SUMMARY

Mastering interactions is a critical skill in any setting and will contribute to a peaceful and prosperous life. After understanding yourself and your context, you will want to analyze those who play a role in your life. We discern between four groups, and each group requires our attention: Indifferent, Neutral, Positive, and Negative. The first two groups, the observers, need our respect and gracious behavior. Group three requires our mindfulness so that we can remain in our power. Group four can be challenging but is a rich source for self-growth, handled in the right way. We learn anger management best with Group 4, as they provide us with anger-inducing incidents the most. Learn from them but stay safe as well.

9

UNDERSTAND WHY YOU ARE ANGRY AND WHAT YOU CAN DO ABOUT IT

“The most intense conflicts, if overcome, leave behind a sense of security and calm that is not easily disturbed.”

— *CARL JUNG*

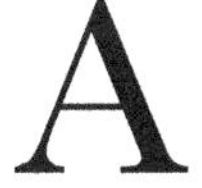

s we can see, sources of anger are manifold. Anger can stem from:

- you and the life you have led so far
- inconsistencies in your context
- the people around you, intentionally and unintentionally

Therefore, there is no simple answer to why you are angry; instead, anger is an invitation to investigate, find the answer, and formulate a plan.

This book offers you a shortcut and a well-trodden path to understanding your anger and yourself as a byproduct. As we slowly eliminate confusion, inconsistencies, and falsehoods from our lives, there will be fewer opportunities for anger. We do not want to eliminate our anger, as it is our friend, protector, and helper. Instead, we want to manage its effect in interactions with others while learning about ourselves.

Challenge yourself to work through this book in three months and resolve at least one identified conflict and its related incidents in the following three months. Document your mood daily to notice the result of your diligent work. It will pay off noticeably and get easier with time.

10

CASE STUDY: CASSIE'S ANGER

"Education is not the learning of facts, but the training of minds to think."

— *ALBERT EINSTEIN*

(N*ames and facts are fictitious)*

Cassie is a 35-year-old marketing manager who works in a highly technical industry. This is a new job for her; she has been in this role and company for nine months. Cassie has a desk job and manages a multi-functional interdisciplinary team of ten co-workers. Only three members report to her directly. She is dependent on her team because each team member's work feeds into the joint team deliverables—the quality of which determines Cassie's reputation.

In the Myers-Briggs test (MBTI), Cassie tested as an INTJ (The Mastermind, The Architect). She is intelligent, keenly process- and goal-oriented, and brilliant at marketing; therefore, she has become one of the youngest managers to handle one of the company's core products. Cassie likes knowing the truth of the matter and is known for creating marketing and branding strategies that work. She is brutally honest and does not typically use tact to appease her co-workers in stressful situations.

People say she has an anger problem, and this perception is slowly defining her reputation, but Cassie can always explain why it was essential to act in the way she did. Usually, it is when she experiences others' negligence toward the quality of their work as a team, which is the highest priority for her. Some have started complaining about her hurtful over-assertiveness, first to onlookers and later to management. The team is now defensive towards her.

Cassie is in a deja vu situation, as she left her last position to escape an almost identical set of circumstances. To make matters worse, she has two toddlers under five who often keep her awake at night. It certainly doesn't help that she is in a continuous state of fatigue.

When she came to me, we resolved to look at her so-called "anger problem" holistically and break the cycle, after a deep dive into her world by using the STOP! -1-2-3 model.

As we can see, she identifies as a person who prioritizes the quality of work (her anger trigger) above interactions and relationships, and her reputation is at risk because of her angry outbursts.

INCIDENT AND CONFLICT ANALYSIS

We use the STOP! -1-2-3 model to better understand what is happening in the conflict "Incompetence and Badmouthing" by analyzing a typical incident:

- In short, what happened? *A company client was in a meeting with Cassie and Team Member A (TMA). Cassie had briefed TMA to prepare answers for the questions that the client had sent in beforehand. Cassie's role was to stay in a high-level discussion while TMA provided the details. It became clear that TMA had not prepared for the meeting. Though the meeting went well on the surface, Cassie was fuming. After the meeting, Cassie gave in to her anger and gave TMA her piece of mind. TMA did not feel responsible and denied any responsibility in the incident. Cassie stomped off. TMA joined her office allies to complain about Cassie.*

- Who was the other person? Who else was involved? *Team Member A and client*
- Was there a recurring conflict that led to this incident? *Inability to collaborate with Team Member A successfully*
- Was the matter related to trust, respect, expectations, and boundaries? *Seemingly, to a lack of respect*
- How did the interaction start? A *detailed briefing about expectations and outcomes, some coaching*
- What triggered your anger, and what was your response to it? A *show of incompetence while clients were present; anger and helplessness*
- Did your response ease or exacerbate the situation? *Exacerbate*
- What was your contribution to the incident? *Potentially, over-delegation*
- What was the context contributing to it? *Lack of quality control of skills, processes, and new hires*
- How did they contribute to the incident? *Apparent lack of willingness to listen, take in feedback, and learn*
- How did the interaction end? *The conflict deepened and was not resolved*
- How did you feel about it straight afterward,

and how do you think of it? *Angry and helpless, and now I do not know what to do.*

ANALYSIS: WHO IS CASSIE?

Her base INTJ personality makes Cassie highly analytical and naturally controlling. Typically, outcome quality is the top priority for an INTJ. They also tend to become irritated and angry quickly and tend not to handle emotions well. They can be judgmental, critical of others and themselves, and not welcome a change of plans. This archetype seems to describe Cassie very well.

Testing her personality profile several times, we discovered that she pivots to a different personality under stressful situations. Under stress, her personality type shifts into an ISTJ, the Inspector or Logistician type. ISTJs are similar to INTJs in many ways, but ISTJs tend to be more sceptical of those who are not like them. When INTJs use their intuitive talents, they easily see the true nature of others and are more accepting. Effectiveness matters significantly to ISTJs, who do not accept the human tendency to make mistakes or behavior outside previously conceived norms.

We concluded that she should become aware of her strictness and recognize the ISTJ pivot in such situations. Taking a step back to de-stress and return to her natural INTJ personality will help her to avoid angry outbursts. I asked her to remember that all personality types have limitations and, more often than not, they are unaware of their blind spots. Understanding others and helping them understand the factors that lead to high-quality outcomes is the right thing to do and a step toward greater maturity.

Reputation is an issue already. We can be sure that Cassie's angry outbursts have not gone unnoticed by the four groups of people in her context: Indifferent, Neutral, Positive, and Negative. She will need to rectify the reputation damage over time by not giving in to stress and consistently behaving differently under pressure.

WHAT DOES CASSIE WANT?

Cassie does not feel satisfied with her life—neither work nor family. She feels she comes up short on both sides, but her work life gives her a sense of identity she enjoys. Her values are family, using her intellect to produce high-quality work, achieving work-life balance, sleeping more, and having sufficient free time.

We established that her ego-self was seemingly healthy and reasonable; however, it was undoubtedly driving her life, as we can see in the assessment below. Symptoms of the ego-self in the driver's seat are anger, feelings of helplessness, guilt, emotional instability, and some pride, dread, fear and complaints.

Cassie's Ego-Self Test

Statements that point to the ego-self running your life. Answer with yes, no, and yes/no.

- *You are proud of yourself and your achievements; you frequently look down on others:* ***yes/no***
- *You talk over others and think you know all the answers:* ***no***
- *You are envious of what others possess:* ***no***
- *You tend to be judgmental and want to minimize the achievements of others:* ***no***
- *You can quickly get angry and even go into a rage;* ***angry, yes / rage, no.***
- *You have an underlying feeling of dread and anxiety. You have many fears:* ***yes/no***
- *You feel helpless and powerless to change your situation:* ***yes***
- *You feel guilty and think you are not doing enough:* ***yes***
- *You have low self-esteem. People can easily shame you; take advantage of you:* ***no***

- *You feel despair and self-doubt, and you do not know your worth:* ***yes/no***
- *You frequently complain about life circumstances:* ***yes/no***
- *Others trigger you quickly, and you have frequent emotional ups and downs:* ***yes***

I recommended a short daily meditation before and after work to process stressful events and the feelings that arise in order to help her become more aware of her wise non-ego-self (higher self). The goals are to let the non-ego-self manage all daily actions and to reach and maintain peace of mind, feelings of courage, neutrality, usefulness, reason, and love. Since her daily schedule with small children does not allow her the luxury of a sitting meditation, we decided on a walking meditation on her way to work after she had dropped off her kids at the daycare facility. We analyzed potential ego-self projections but couldn't identify any. I specifically asked Cassie if she felt her work input is low quality. It was not the case, so we ruled out a projection.

Cassie worries that she cannot yet feel and think simultaneously, on her feet. However, she avoided a recent anger outburst successfully. When an incident happened while we were conducting her deep dive self-exploration, she realized that our discussions had helped her stay aware and not give in to the irritation she was feeling. She also learned to direct her attention toward what she wanted to achieve with the team, and focus less on her team's shortcomings.

WHAT IS CASSIE'S CONTEXT?

Cassie doesn't fit in. I advised her to think about a potential workplace change in the long run, as we had analyzed her context's MVP using the deep dive methodology and discovered six challenges.

Cassie's Context Culture

Based on HOGAN's 10 MVPs (motivations, values, and preferences), evaluate the culture of your context. Answer with yes, no, or yes/no:

Recognition: being known, seen, visible, famous

- Do you value recognition? ***no***
- Do the leaders in your context value recognition? ***no***

Power: challenge, competition, achievement, and success

- Do you value power? ***no***
- Do the leaders in your context value power? ***no***

Hedonism: fun, excitement, variety, and pleasure

- Do you value hedonism? ***yes***
- Do the leaders in your context value hedonism? ***no***

Altruistic: serving others and helping the less fortunate

- Do you value altruism? ***yes***
- Do the leaders in your context value altruism? ***no***

Affiliation: frequent and varied social contact

- Do you value affiliation? ***yes***
- Do the leaders in your context value affiliation? ***no***

Tradition: morality, family values, and devotion to duty

- Do you value tradition? ***yes***
- Do the leaders in your context value tradition? ***no***

Security: structure, order, and predictability

- Do you value security? ***yes***
- Do the leaders in your context value security? ***no***

Commerce: earning money, realizing profits, finding opportunities

- Do you value commerce? ***no***
- Do the leaders in your context value commerce? ***yes***

Aesthetics: the look, feel, and design of products and artistic work

- Do you value aesthetics? ***yes***
- Do the leaders in your context value aesthetics? ***yes***

Science: new ideas, technology, and rational problem-solving

- Do you value science? ***yes***
- Do the leaders in your context value science? ***no***

We reflected on the cultural values and summarized our findings:

- What mismatches do you see? *Many mismatches.*
- What does that mean to you? *This may not be the best long-term workplace for Cassie.*
- What are your insights and conclusions of the evaluation? *Cassie needs a workplace that values quality and science highly.*

Secondly, we looked at the "rules of the game" in her context and discovered more shortcomings (see below). Yes, there are ways to cope, but this environment will not be suitable for her in the long run.

Cassie's Insights regarding Rules of the Game in her Context

- What are the 5-10 rules in your context? *Keep your head down, never complain, produce good work, and do not waste company resources.*
- Which rules are acceptable to you? *Cassie would like to discuss aspects of the work process that aren't working. However, her boss interprets her continuous striving for higher quality as complaints.*
- Which rules irritate you and make you angry? *Never complain; keep your head down. This is difficult when there are recurring quality issues.*

- If so, is there a way to decrease the sense of irritation? *No, not being able to express my thoughts and improve the quality of work outcomes is painful.*
- What else do you notice? *With meditation and coaching, I can use my irritation to trigger growth and self-development.*
- What is your conclusion? *I will need to accept that it is the way it is, for now.*

Key Players in Cassie's Work Context

- Who are the 5-10 key players who define your context? *Ten team members, my boss, the department head, and the HR representative.*
- What are they passionate about? What do they value? *Having no tension and conflicts, business as planned, business outcomes*
- What are their goals? *A 2-year plan, agenda, and goals are not well communicated and unclear.*
- Do the key players have a joint vision? What is it? *No, there is noticeable tension in the leadership team regarding the future.*
- What is your ambition in this context? Do you want to be a top player? *No, there is no way that I can be. I do not feel that I belong.*

We listed the people in Cassie's circle, and we spread them across four groups, discerning how she felt about them. We identified five positive influences that helped her to enjoy her work, and three challenging ones.

People Cassie Interacts with Regularly in her Workplace

We identified 19 people in her context.

1) Name of the person: *boss*

Indifferent (1), neutral (2), positive (3), or negative (4)? *negative*

2) Name of the person:*department head*

Indifferent (1), neutral (2), positive (3), or negative (4)? *positive*

3) Name of the person: *HR representative*

Indifferent (1), neutral (2), positive (3), or negative (4)? *positive*

4) Name of the person: *10 team members*

Indifferent (1), neutral (2), positive (3), or negative (4)?

5 neutral

3 positive

2 negative

5) Name of the person:*6 observers*

Indifferent (1), neutral (2), positive (3), or negative (4)? *indifferent*

Current Active Conflicts in Cassie's Context

We identified three currently active conflicts in her workplace.

Name of conflict: *Incompetence and Badmouthing*

- Name of the person involved: *team member A*
- Are others involved? *two of team member A's friends*
- Age of conflict: *4 month*
- Degree of Stress (Impact on Mood) in %: *90%*
- Typical Triggers: *quality of work*
- Priority for resolution: *Priority 1*

Name of conflict: *Reputation damaging*

- Name of the person involved: *team member B*
- Are others involved? *unsure*
- Age of conflict: *6 months*
- Degree of Stress (Impact on Mood) in %: *60%*
- Typical Triggers: *gossip*
- Priority for resolution: *Priority 3*

Name of conflict: *Miscommunication*

- Name of the person involved: *boss*
- Are others involved? *the leadership team (assumption)*
- Age of conflict: *6 months*
- Degree of Stress (Impact on Mood) in %: *60%*
- Typical Triggers: *inability to improve processes that do not work.*
- Priority for resolution: *2*

IN SUMMARY

Cassie's Analysis Tool: STOP! -1-2-3, the upper half

- **Potential underlying conflict:** *Unresolved issues with Team Member A for four months. The previous resolution offers were unsuccessful.*
- **Context:** *workplace*
- **Incident:** *Meeting with client went wrong, anger episode*
- **Your name:** *Cassie*
- **Their name:** *Team Member A*
- **Others involved:** *Client, Team Member A's friends*
- **Trigger:** *Cassie cannot control her anger when quality is at stake (Trigger).*

- ***Response:*** Anger and helplessness
- ***Your contribution:*** More inner work is required.
- ***The context's contribution:*** *The context will remain as is; optimization is not possible.*
- ***Their contribution:*** *Seemingly doesn't respect Cassie and her instructions. Potential lack of social skills and other skills, immaturity, or intentional sabotage? Team Member A is a question mark.*
- ***Significant details:*** *Team Member A is unable to collaborate and seemingly doesn't respect Cassie and her instructions. Discussions with Cassie's boss about improving the work process remain fruitless. This company doesn't seem to prioritize optimizing social skills and developing new hires. Therefore, escalating the solution for the incident to the boss is not possible.*

Cassie's Solution Design Tool: STOP! -1-2-3, the lower half

Your Contribution to the Incident (1):

- *Not enough preparation*
- *Unclear values and priorities*
- *Potential lack of communication, process, and quality management, and not enough negotiation with the boss*

The Contribution of the Context to the Incident (2)

Context: *workplace*

- *Lack of follow-up*
- *Unclear responsibilities*
- *Potential sub-par process*

Their Contribution to the Incident (3)

- *Lack of skill or knowledge*
- *Unclear picture of abilities*
- *Unclear development plan for the junior co-worker*

Solution Goals

- **Self-development & -growth:** *Integrate meditation, self-reflection, awareness of triggers, and maintain a healthy lifestyle. Improve the ability to stay calm and not react. Answer the question: How long do I want to remain in this company?*
- ***Preventing future incidents:*** *Better preparation, less delegation*
- **Complete curing of the conflict** (20-30% of cases):/
- **Rehabilitating the relationship** (5-10% of cases): /
- **Mitigation, moderation, and coping (5-10% of**

cases): *Keeping diplomatic distance from Boss and Team Member A*

Solution Strategy

- ***Avoidance: Doing nothing.***

Solution Plan

- ***Position:*** *Take a step back.*
- ***Goals & Strategy:*** 3 chosen goals of *self-development, prevention, and coping. Avoidance strategy*
- ***Implementation Plan:*** *Self-focused*
- ***Action:*** *Meditation and fitness rituals, self-reflection*
- ***Refinement*** *(WIP)*
- ***Control:*** *Exercising self-empowerment, mindful awareness*

We concluded that Cassie's hands were tied in this conflict, because there was no way to resolve the four-month-old dispute under these circumstances. A sign pointing to this was her feelings of helplessness and confusion. She had given her power away to the circumstances. Therefore, we chose an avoidance strategy so she could take the time to invest energy in herself. Choosing to step back and accept the situation is a self-empowering move. The choice to suffer or not to suffer was hers. She is also aware of preventive measures she can apply, for example, delegating fewer tasks to Team Member A. In the future, aspects of the context may shift, and her boss and TMA may have a change of heart. However, Cassie is not waiting for this to happen. She decided to let go. Cassie has taken back her power and stepped out of the conflict by focusing on herself and doing her best every day. Conflicts and resulting incidents need at least two emotionally participating parties to survive. The paradigm shift in her mind will also reduce her triggers' potency. She will learn not to react when similar incidents happen, but rather respond to what is happening consciously. She left with a happy smile and lightness in her step because she had resolved the issue in her mind. Everything else can remain as is.

LEAVE A REVIEW!

Customer Reviews

2

5.0 out of 5 stars

5 star		100%
4 star		0%
3 star		0%
2 star		0%
1 star		0%

See all verified purchase reviews ›

Share your thoughts with other customers

Write a customer review

If you enjoyed this book, do leave a 1-Click review. I would be incredibly thankful if you take just 60 seconds to write a brief review, even if it is a few sentences.

►Scan the QR code below to leave a review!◄

CONCLUSIONS

> *"Wholeness is not achieved by cutting off a portion of one's being, but by the integration of the contraries."*
>
> — CARL JUNG

I hope, dear Reader, that you have found your anger cure with this book. I hope you feel empowered and armed well enough to be able to tackle any anger incident you face. Managing your anger will undoubtedly benefit you in all areas of your life. When you begin to see your anger as a friend and the sign of a deeper problem, it becomes a helper and guide to help you shift your thought patterns. Analyzing each incident and trigger will bring you closer to your wise non-ego self, step-by-step. It is an exciting adventure.

The book has provided you with a simple three-step formula for anger management: The STOP! -1-2-3 Analysis and the Solution Design. The self-investigation and soul-searching in preparation for anger management require some heavy lifting. Instead of complaining about others and life circumstances, we commit to investing our time in understanding ourselves more—it is a swap that promises greater peace of mind.

After reading and working through this book, assess your outcome by asking yourself the following questions:

- Do I know myself and what I want better than I did before?
- Do I better understand my current situation?
- Am I able to anticipate future incidents that could potentially trigger me, and stop automatically reacting to triggers?
- Do I see where I stand and what my next step could be?
- Do I know how to use whatever trigger or incident that shows up in my life to increase my awareness, sense of self, and resilience?

All of your answers should be yes; otherwise, go back and work through whatever is still unclear again. Good luck!

If you enjoyed this book, dear Reader, go to www.zarminapenner.com and find out more.

11

WORKBOOK: BLANK TEMPLATES

N*ote: The following templates are available for download on www.zarminapenner.com.*

ANGER INCIDENT: INITIAL QUESTIONS TO ASK YOURSELF

Describe the incident and tell the story.

- In short, what happened?
- Who was the other person? Who else was involved?
- Was there a recurring conflict that led to this incident?
- Was the matter related to trust, respect, expectations, and boundaries?

- How did the interaction start?
- What triggered your anger, and what was your response to it?
- Did your response ease or exacerbate the situation?
- What was your contribution to the incident?
- What was the context contributing to it?
- How did they contribute to the incident?
- How did the interaction end?
- How did you feel about it immediately afterward, and how do you think of it?

ANALYSIS TOOL

Now read your story and summarize your analysis findings in brief as best as you can:

- Incident:
- Your name:
- Their name:
- Others involved:
- Potential underlying conflict:
- Your contribution:
- The context's contribution:
- Their contribution:
- Significant details:

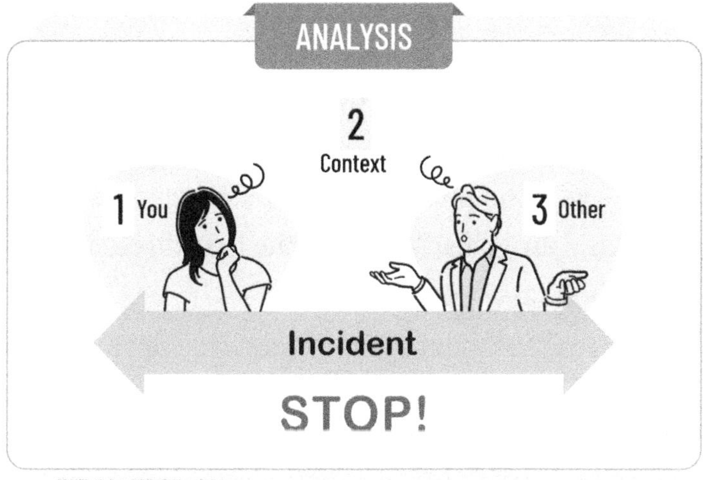

Image 7: The 1-2-3-Stop! Mental Model and Process: Analysis

SOLUTION DESIGN TOOL

With your analysis findings, choose your Solution Goals (as many as you deem necessary) from the five potential goals depicted in the image. What do you want to achieve with the analysis findings and your learnings?

Choose one solution strategy from the three possible strategies depicted in the image.

- Your Solution Goals:
- Your Solution Strategy:

Then design your Solution Plan:

- What is your position on this incident, your starting point?
- How will you implement your strategy and reach your goals? What are the first three steps you will take?

Let it sit for a while, and then take action. With each step, refine your plan of action. Your ultimate goal is to control the situation by behaving differently and preventing future incidents from happening. The gift of the anger incident is the learning and growth you achieve from it.

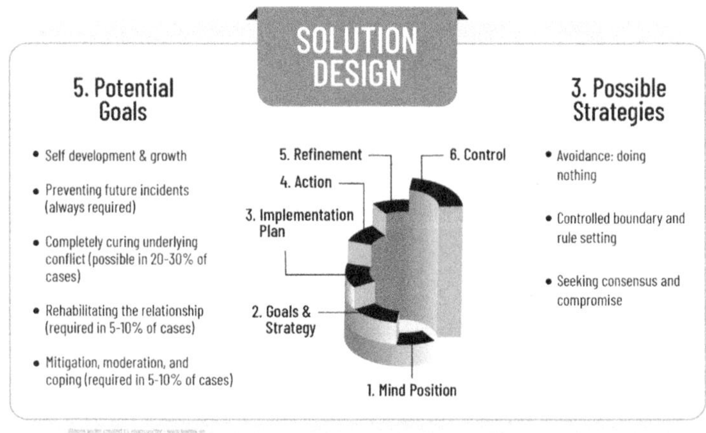

Image 8: The 1-2-3-Stop! Mental Model and Process: Solution Design

YOUR IDENTITY, REPUTATION, AND PERSONALITY

Refer to the instructions in the book.

Describe your identity:

✎...

✎...

Describe your reputation, potentially with tests findings:

✎...

✎...

Describe your personality, with test findings:

✎...

✎...

YOUR PRIMARY FIVE VALUES

Refer to the instructions in the book and describe the current five values that relate to your non-ego-self:

Value 1:

✎...

Value 2:

✎...

Value 3:

✎...

Value 4:

✎...

Value 5:

✎...

TEST YOUR VALUES

Ego-self test: Please evaluate with yes, no, or yes/no.

Statements that point to the ego-self running your life

- *You are proud of yourself and your achievements; you frequently look down on others.*
- *You talk over others and think you know all the answers.*
- *You are envious of what others possess.*
- *You tend to be judgmental and want to minimize the achievements of others.*
- *You can quickly get angry and even go into a rage.*

- *You have an underlying feeling of dread and anxiety. You have many fears.*
- *You feel helpless and powerless to change your situation.*
- *You feel guilty and think you are not doing enough.*
- *You have low self-esteem. People can easily shame you and take advantage of you.*
- *You feel despair and self-doubt, and you do not know your own worth.*
- *You frequently complain about life circumstances.*
- *Others trigger you quickly, and you have frequent emotional ups and downs.*

YOU AND YOUR CONTEXT CULTURE

Based on HOGAN's 10 MVPs (motivations, values, and preferences), evaluate the culture of your context. Answer with yes, no, or yes/no:

Recognition: being known, seen, visible, famous

- Do you value recognition?
- Do the leaders in your context value recognition?

Power: challenge, competition, achievement, and success

- Do you value power?
- Do the leaders in your context value power?

Hedonism: fun, excitement, variety, and pleasure

- Do you value hedonism?
- Do the leaders in your context value hedonism?

Altruistic: serving others and helping the less fortunate

- Do you value altruism?
- Do the leaders in your context value altruism?

Affiliation: frequent and varied social contact

- Do you value affiliation?
- Do the leaders in your context value affiliation?

Tradition: morality, family values, and devotion to duty

- Do you value tradition?
- Do the leaders in your context value tradition?

Security: structure, order, and predictability

- Do you value security?
- Do the leaders in your context value security?

Commerce: earning money, realizing profits, finding opportunities

- Do you value commerce?
- Do the leaders in your context value commerce?

Aesthetics: the look, feel, and design of products and artistic work

- Do you value aesthetics?
- Do the leaders in your context value aesthetics?

Science: new ideas, technology, and rational problem-solving

- Do you value science?
- Do the leaders in your context value science?

Now reflect on the comparison of the cultural values and summarize your findings:

- What mismatches do you see?

✎...

- What does this mean to you?

✎...

- What are your insights and conclusions of the evaluation?

✎...

RULES OF THE GAME IN YOUR CONTEXT

Identify the apparent and hidden rules of the game in your context:

- What are the 5-10 rules in your context?

✎...

✎...

✎...

✎...

✎...

- Which rules are acceptable to you?

✎...

✎...

- Which rules irritate you and make you angry?

✎...

✎...

- If so, is there a way to decrease the sense of irritation?

✎...

✎...

- What else do you notice?

✎...

✎...

- What is your conclusion?

✎...

✎...

KEY PLAYERS IN YOUR CONTEXT

Identify the key players in your context:

Name the context:

- Who are the 5-10 key players who define your context?

✎...

✎...

✎...

✎...

✎...

- What are they passionate about? What do they value?

✎...

✎...

- What are their goals?

✎...

✎...

- Do the key players have a joint vision? What is it?

✎...

✎...

- What is your ambition in this context? Do you want to be a top player?

✎...

✎...

PEOPLE YOU INTERACT WITHIN YOUR CONTEXT

Identify the ten people you interact with most in your context:

Name the context:

1) Name of the person:

Indifferent (1), neutral (2), positive (3), or negative (4)?

2) Name of the person:

Indifferent (1), neutral (2), positive (3), or negative (4)?

3) Name of the person:

Indifferent (1), neutral (2), positive (3), or negative (4)?

4) Name of the person:

Indifferent (1), neutral (2), positive (3), or negative (4)?

5) Name of the person:

Indifferent (1), neutral (2), positive (3), or negative (4)?

6) Name of the person:

Indifferent (1), neutral (2), positive (3), or negative (4)?

7) Name of the person:

Indifferent (1), neutral (2), positive (3), or negative (4)?

8) Name of the person:

Indifferent (1), neutral (2), positive (3), or negative (4)?

9) Name of the person:

Indifferent (1), neutral (2), positive (3), or negative (4)?

10) Name of the person:

Indifferent (1), neutral (2), positive (3), or negative (4)?

CURRENTLY ACTIVE CONFLICTS IN YOUR CONTEXT

Identify your three currently active conflicts in this context:

Name the context:

Name of conflict:

- Name of the person involved:
- Are others involved?
- Age of conflict:
- Degree of Stress (Impact on Mood) in %:
- Typical Triggers
- Priority for resolution:

Name of conflict:

- Name of the person involved:
- Are they indifferent (1), neutral (2), positive (3), or negative (4)?
- Are others involved?
- Age of conflict:
- Degree of Stress (Impact on Mood) in %:
- Typical Triggers
- Priority for resolution:

Name of conflict:

- Name of the person involved:
- Are they indifferent (1), neutral (2), positive (3), or negative (4)?
- Are others involved?
- Age of conflict:
- Degree of Stress (Impact on Mood) in %:
- Typical Triggers
- Priority for resolution:

CURRENTLY ACTIVE CONFLICTS WITH NEGATIVES

Here are questions to ask dealing with Group four (negatives):

1. Are they earnestly considering your proposal(s) for a solution?

✎...

2.Do they listen carefully and respond?

✎...

3.Are they kind to you in behavior and words?

✎...

4.Do they respect you and your boundaries?

✎...

5.Do they accept responsibility for the incident or conflict?

✎...

6.Are they able to control their emotions?

✎...

7. Do they show remorse and try to change their ways after the conversation?

✎...

8.Does the interaction feel right? What does your gut feeling say?

✎...

A FREE GIFT FOR OUR READERS

To best prepare for the book, use this guide to identify your anger triggers quickly!

Just scan the QR code below!

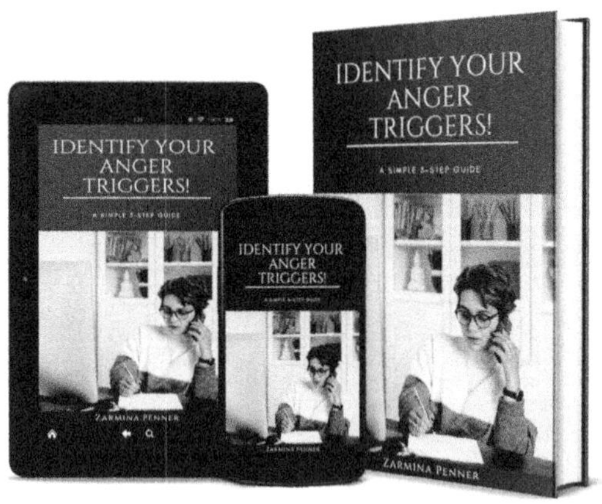

RESOURCES

Ekman, P. (2015). *Emotions revealed: understanding faces and feeling* (Chinese Edition) (1st ed.). Hunan Science and Technology Press.

Ekman, P. E. (n.d.). *What are emotions?* Paulekman.Com. Retrieved March 26, 2022, from https://www.paulekman.com/universal-emotions/

Hawkins, D. R., MD Ph.D. (2012). *Power vs. force: The hidden determinants of human behavior* (1st ed.). Veritas Publishing.

Hogan Assessments. (2021, May 25). Flash Report. https://www.hoganassessments.com/reports/flash-report/

Hogan, R. (2006). *Personality and the fate of organizations* (1st ed.). Routledge.

Hosford, A. H., & Ashcroft, C. A. (2010). *Moodscope - Lift your mood with a little help from your friends.* Https://Www.Moodscope.Com/. Retrieved March 27, 2022, from https://www.moodscope.com/

Joel Mark Witt, J. M. W., & Antonia Dodge, A. D. (n.d.). *Genius style assessment.* Personality Hacker. Retrieved March 27, 2022, from https://personalityhacker.com/genius-personality-test/

NERIS Analytics Limited. (2011). *Free personality test.* 16Personalities. https://www.16personalities.com/free-personality-test

Oxford Languages and Google - English | Oxford Languages. (2021, December 2). https://languages.oup.com/Google-Dictionary-En/

Rosenberg, R. R. (2018). *The human magnet syndrome: The codependent narcissist trap.* Morgan James Publishing.

Simon, G. S. K. (2010). *In sheep's clothing: Understanding and dealing with manipulative people* (First Edition, 2nd Edition, second edition is exclusive to Parkhurst Brothers pub ed.). Parkhurst Brothers Publishers Inc.

Singer, M. A. (2013). *The untethered soul: The journey beyond yourself* (Gift Edition w/ Ribbon Marker ed.). New Harbinger Publications.

Wikipedia contributors. (2022, March 21). *Higher self*. Wikipedia. https://en.wikipedia.org/wiki/Higher_self

ABOUT THE AUTHOR

After recognizing her passion for aligning organizations and teams with their vision and goals and helping business professionals live their best lives, Zarmina Penner, a medical doctor by training, moved into business consulting and executive coaching over 20 years ago. Her work is, in essence, about providing practical solutions for professional and personal everyday concerns, building high-spirited collaborative communities and teams, and inspiring others to think differently. She works in English and German and lives near Frankfurt, Germany. For more information, visit www.zarminapenner.com.

NOTES

2. UNDERSTAND ANGER

1. Ekman, P. (2015). Emotions Revealed: Understanding Faces and Feeling (Chinese Edition) (1st ed.). Hunan Science and Technology Press.
2. Hawkins, D. R., MD PhD. (2012). *Power vs. Force: The Hidden Determinants of Human Behavior* (1st ed.). Veritas Publishing.

5. UNDERSTAND WHAT YOU WANT

1. The Untethered Soul: The Journey Beyond Yourself, Michael A. Singer (2007)

8. UNDERSTAND YOUR ACTIVE CONFLICTS AND RELATED INCIDENTS

1. Rosenberg, R. R. (2018). The Human Magnet Syndrome: The Codependent Narcissist Trap. Morgan James Publishing.
2. Simon, G. S. K. (2010). *In Sheep's Clothing: Understanding and Dealing with Manipulative People* (First Edition, 2nd Edition, second edition is exclusive to Parkhurst Brothers pub ed.). Parkhurst Brothers Publishers Inc.

Made in the USA
Las Vegas, NV
29 August 2022

54288766R00090